MAKING THEM MISS:

THE SWEET SCIENCE OF BOXING

By: Joseph "Bruza" Johnson

Copyright 2018 by Joseph Johnson

ISBN: 9798734676585

Contact The Author

Email – JoeJohnson0582@gmail.com
Facebook - Joseph Johnson
Twitter – Joseph Johnson
Instagram – @Bruza_F_Ladies

Book Production - Crystell Publications
We Help You Self-Publish Your Book
405-414-3991
CrystellPublications.com

Dedication

This book is dedicated to the loving memory of my Grandmother, Ena Johnson and my mother, Ovita Johnson. May they Rest in Paradise.

To my daughter Nicole, Daddy will always love you.

CONTENTS

FORWARD

"Health is wealth and knowledge is power."

It is said that with great power comes great responsibility. The responsibility to not only think for yourself, but also for others. The power of knowledge in any specialized area is called a skill. With a skill set such as boxing, you will gain the knowledge and the ability to manipulate the fight. You will be able to make an opponent move in the direction that you choose, therefore influencing their attacks while simultaneously setting them up for your counterattacks.

You are fully responsible for any encounter that you may find yourself in, even if you are attacked. If you lose or get hurt in combat it is due to poor preparation on your behalf, and if you should hurt or injure an opponent, you are also liable.

When you master the sweet science of boxing, you must show restraint. You must exercise discipline in a way that's similar to kicking a habit. You trained your skill to be second nature, now you must exercise the restraint to not use it at all.

INTRODUCTION

Since the beginning of my boxing career, I've been looking for an instructional boxing guide, one that would give me boxing tips. I never found one. The only books that I have found on boxing were autobiographies, biographies, and workouts.

My boxing career started at the age of 17. I am now 36 years of age. My book, *Making Them Miss: The Sweet Science of Boxing,* was created to keep your game on track and not your wig pushed back. This is a book for those who are interested in the craft but may not have the funds to pay a top-notch trainer or highly reputable gym.

CHAPTER 1

SUCCESS

Proper preparation + Opportunity = Success

Elite athletes don't train in seasons, they train year-round. You will become a good athlete by training within your season. However, an elite athlete will make a good athlete look like an amateur.

Some examples:

Sugar Ray vs. Haglar

Mike Tyson vs. Frank Bruno

Roy Jones vs. Trinidad

Mayweather vs. Cotto

Opportunity is spontaneous. In order to be prepared for opportunity, one must stay abreast.

Train when your opponent is training. Train when your opponent is resting. Train all year long.

CHAPTER 2

DISCIPLINE

Discipline in boxing is the practice of solely using your hands. No kicks. No grabs. No knees. No elbows. No matter how frustrated one gets, you must find a way to achieve your goal with your fist.

Discipline is the practice that governs our actions and reactions. Strengthen your discipline for a more effective craft.

CHAPTER 3

FIGHTING STANCE

Assuming that you are right-handed, your right hand is your power hand. Find a full-size mirror or something in which you can clearly see your reflection. Stand in front of your mirror with your body straight, and your feet shoulder-width apart. Take a step back, about a foot straight back, with your right leg. Turn your feet with your body to a 45-degree angle to your right. This should place you in a sideways position in front of your mirror.

In a calf-raised position, stand on the ball of your feet. Slightly bend at the knee and hip in a slight sitting position. Although sideways, your head should remain forward, facing the mirror. Chin tucked down toward your chest, with your left cheek touching your left shoulder. Eyes always up. Keep your fists on the sides of your face just beneath your eyes. Elbows down. Arms pressed against your body. Teeth clenched at all times. This is the orthodox stance.

If you are left-handed, do this toward your left-hand side. This is the southpaw stance. Remain in your fighting stance for as long as you can, until you get comfortable with it. While in front of your mirror, get used to what this position looks like from head to toe. Repeat until you get comfortable. This is your fighting stance.

CHAPTER 4

BREATHING

Condition Your Breathing To Expand Your Lungs And Increase Your Stamina. If You Can't Breathe, Then You Can't Fight. In Any Sport Or Activity, The One Who Wins Or Dominates Is Usually The One With The Best Stamina. This Is True In Football, Basketball, Soccer, Track & Field, And Especially Boxing. An Unskilled Fighter Can Outlast And Win Over An Expert If The Expert Has Poor Stamina.

Oxygen is the element that fuels your muscles, and poor circulation will leave your muscles fatigued. The more muscles you use, the more oxygen is needed to keep those muscles working. So if you can't breathe, then you can't fight.

Practice taking a deep breath through your nose before executing your combination. Exhale small amounts of air with each punch through clenched teeth.

When boxing, your abdominal muscles should be flexed at all times. Exhaling while contracting your abdominals will make your core muscles contract even more.

Breathing is a privilege, exercise it!

CHAPTER 5

SPRINTING

Cardio is an important tool in any sport, if you can't breathe then you can't participate. In boxing, the one who does his road work will do whatever he wants in the ring, while the guy who doesn't will only do what he can.

For athletes, one of the oldest forms of cardio is jogging. Jogging is an excellent way to lose weight and build stamina, amidst having several other benefits. Jogging will give you the stamina to box 12 rounds.

Sprinting is taking your road work to the next level. There will come a time when you won't need to make weight, and your stamina will be on high. This doesn't mean that your road work is complete. This simply means that now you can focus your road work in the direction of the fight.

A fight may start off slow and explode spontaneously. Sprinting is the intense cardiovascular training for the spontaneous outburst in a fight.

Sprinting will allow you to breeze through an intense fight. Build a tolerance for high intensity and you will be able to fight stronger for longer. In addition to jogging and doing your road work, complete no less than 100-yard dash sprints for every minute you intend to fight.

Jogging will help you cruise through the fight.

Sprinting will help you brawl through the fight.

The jump rope will aid your footwork through the fight.

CHAPTER 6

FOOTWORK

Footwork wins fights! Your feet take you to the fight and also carry you away from the fight. Each step within arm's reach of an opponent should be accompanied by a jab. It is important for the speed of your feet to match the speed of your punches, as you should be quick to punch. Good footwork brings about good offense, and defense, as it allows you to work different angles. Footwork techniques such as the pivot step, sidestep, diagonal back step, and the pedal step can give you a major edge over your competition.

Pivoting is simply sweeping your back foot behind your leading leg while turning at a 45-degree angle. If performed correctly you'll flank your opponent. Offensively, pivoting should be performed after the last punch is thrown in your combination. Defensively, pivoting is effective after evading a punch, like after a slip and roll.

A sidestep is simply stepping from one side to the

next, like stepping left or right. The sidestep will throw off the direction or angle of your opponent's attack. Pivoting maybe applied when sidestepping in the direction of your leading leg.

Backstepping should always be performed diagonally. Never step straight back. Step back at an angle to offset your opponent's direction. If you step straight back as your opponent proceeds forward, they will remain on top of you if their step is greater than yours.

The pedal step is a slight step back with your leading foot, followed by a forward step with your back foot. A pedal step will help you move out of the way quickly and can be applied after a pivot step to place you back in position.

Example:

In a left foot leading stance, slip right, evading the jab. Then slip left evading the power hand. Pivot step to your left, placing yourself on the right-hand side of your opponent. Shoot your combination while facing your opponent's side, then pedal step to the front of your opponent. Shoot another combination, then back step diagonally with the jab.

CHAPTER 7

RHYTHM

Whether you realize it or not, life moves to a rhythm. The ocean moves to a rhythm. Birds fly to a rhythm. The earth spins to a rhythm. A boxer also fights to a rhythm. Find your rhythm! Your rhythm will be a steady pace that you can perform effortlessly. Start slow, and once perfected, you can increase your speed. More often than not you will find this pace when fatigued.

The rhythm of your hands and feet should be in unison. Every twist and step you make should be in harmony with your offense or defense. A boxer's rhythm is very similar to a waltz or ballroom dance.

When moving forward, step with your leading leg than your back leg. When moving backward, step with your back leg than your front leg. When stepping to the right side, right leg first. When stepping to the left side, left leg first. Make sure to never crisscross your legs or step beyond your other foot in front of your opponent.

Always keep a distance of about 12 inches between feet, never closer.

Exercise:

Step on a small trampoline, or a large car tire without a rim. In your fighting stance, bounce back and forth on the balls of your feet. This is called distributing weight.

Dance on your opponents with your footwork and frequently change up your rhythm.

CHAPTER 8

YOUR CORE

A boxer's primary muscles are legs, back, shoulders, forearms, calves, and core. Out of these muscles, the core has got to be the most important, as it protects your internal organs.

Many people refer to the abdomen as the core when the core also consists of the obliques and the lower back. Picture a big rubber band wrapping around your midsection. This is your core. The innermost core muscle is responsible for holding your internal organs in place. Its functions are twisting motions. On top of these muscles are your obliques. Your obliques run across your core diagonally. Its functions are side to side and diagonal flexion. On top of your obliques are your abdominal muscles. These muscles run from underneath your chest into your pelvic area. Its function is vertical flexion.

The core is of major importance both offensively and defensively. Strengthening your core adds speed to your slips and punches while building endurance. Every punch, except for the jab, starts with a twist of the core. Strengthen these muscles to make your punches stronger and faster.

If your opponent is faster than you are, shots to the core will slow them down.

CHAPTER 9

KEEP YOUR HEAD MOVING

Your brain is the central nervous system of your body. Stop the head and you stop the body. Your brain is responsible for all of your body's motor functions, so protect your head at all costs. Side-to-side head motions, called slips, while in front of an opponent, will cause them to slow down their attack while trying to time your movement. Keep your movements unpredictable by adding combinations while in motion.

Example:

In an orthodox stance, slip right while moving away from your opponent's power hand. Then slip left while moving back toward their power hand. Now slip right while popping the left jab. Slip left while swinging the right hook. Slip right while firing the left uppercut. Then back out with the jab or a pivot step.

Each time you stand in front of your opponent, change the number of head movements before your attack and also change up your combinations.

CHAPTER 10

DEFENSE OVER OFFENSE

"Protect yourself at all times."

This is the most important rule in boxing. Unlike most sports, where you're on offense one turn then defense the next, when boxing you're on offense and defense at the same time, all the time. Keep your hands up to protect your head. Stay on your toes to keep your movements fast.

The sweet science of boxing is to hit without getting hit, but in order to do so, you must train your body to work in unison. You must train your foot speed to be just as fast as your hands. Also, your slips and ducks must be as fast as one's hands to be effective.

A strong defense is dominant over a strong offense any day. If you can't touch me, then you can't beat me.

CHAPTER 11

TRAIN YOUR EYES

"Use your eyes, there not just supposed to be hazel, they supposed to do some work around here."

-Money Mike

Some people have a habit of closing their eyes while they swing. Others close their eyes when something is thrown at them. Never take your eyes off your opponent. It's not the punches you see, but the ones you don't see which cause the most damage. For example, knockouts.

Head down. Chin tucked. Eyes up. Follow objects with your eyes, not your head. Hand-eye coordination is a must, so develop it.

Focus mitts are a great way to train your hand-eye coordination.

CHAPTER 12

TIMING

Master the art of time! Learn when a target is most vulnerable. Just because you see an opening doesn't mean it's available to you. An opponent can leave his guard down on purpose, which looks to you as an unprotected area. This could be to get you to throw a specific punch in order to counter your attack. The open target you saw was a setup.

An opponent in full guard must open a target when attacking. Throwing a left jab exposes the left rib cage. Learn to get around the jab, and the left rib cage is your target.

Example:

Slip right of your opponent's left jab while shooting your right uppercut toward their left rib cage.

Two bags in a boxing gym that assist with timing is the speed bag and double end bag. The double end bag is a small bag that hangs from the ceiling and attaches to the floor. This bag has an elastic band that makes it snap back after being struck. The double end bag must be hit or evaded on return; this is the bag that hits back.

The speed bag hangs from a make-shift ceiling and is shaped like a teardrop. The best way to time the speed bag is by sound, as it may move too quickly for the eyes. Count the knocks or bounces. When you hit the speed bag, it will move away from you. This is the first bounce. Moving back toward you is the second bounce. Then away again is the third bounce. Your strike comes after every third bounce. This is when the bag is traveling in your direction.

For perfect timing, keep count in your head. One... Two... Three... Strike!

CHAPTER 13

HAND PROTECTION

In boxing, your hands are your biggest assets, so it is imperative that you keep your hands protected. Here is my method to hand protection.

Grab a few gauze pads, about six to eight. Tape the edges together to bind them. Now make two of these.

Use extra-long or double-length hand wraps to cover the entire hand in one shot. Attach the wrap to your thumb. With fingers spread, wrap the wrist about three times. Make sure it's snug but never tight. Leaving your wrist from the thumb side, wrap around the knuckles twice, then wrap around the hand coming down towards the wrist. Wrap once around the wrist then once around the thumb. Place your gauze pad over the knuckles. Coming from underneath the thumb, bring your wrap between each finger, starting with the pinky. Then come around the bottom of the thumb, then back around the knuckles three more times. Once again around the wrist, then cover the hand coming downward. Fasten at the wrist.

There are different methods to wrap the hands, find a method that works for you.

CHAPTER **14**

AIM

The smaller the target, the more accurate the aim. Don't aim for the face, pick a body part on the face. Aim your protruding knuckle at the chin, a tooth, or the bridge of the nose. Pick an eye or an ear and punch through it.

Draw bright circles on your heavy bag and attack them with your protruding knuckles. Hang up a string or rope for aim when shadowboxing.

CHAPTER 15

HOW TO HIT

You must commit to the act. Go all the way and never hesitate. Hitting is an act of violence, so hitting with bad intentions is more effective as you will aim for more vital targets. Don't just hit, but punch through your opponents.

The most effective way to punch is by using your protruding knuckles. Make a tight fist. You will have one or two knuckles that are bigger than the rest. These are your strikers. When punching, drive your protruding knuckles into your opponent like a spare. I like to call this "touching the soul". In the boxing world, it's called "digging in the body." An added twist on your punch can be used to cut around the eye of your opponent.

Using your protruding knuckles will knock out teeth. When digging in the body, your opponent can lose control of bodily functions and can end up vomiting, urinating, or defecating. They might also break a few ribs.

Practice punching with your protruding knuckles when shadowboxing, hitting the heavy bag, hitting focus pads, and when sparring.

CHAPTER 16

THE JAB

The jab is the most important punch you have. The jab serves as offense and defense, along with several other jobs. You can offensively advance toward an opponent with the jab, or defensively back away from an opponent with the jab.

The jab is your locator. It helps to measure the distance between you and your target. Using your jab will let you know how far or close you must be to make contact with your opponent. Quick snaps from your jab will keep your opponent at bay. The jab should be executed with a step. This is called stepping into a punch or backing out with a punch. Stepping into a punch cuts off excess space and adds power to your punch. Backing out with the jab prevents your opponent's counterattack and puts distance between you and your opponent after you release a combination.

Your jab should be thrown quickly, and retracted just as fast, putting you back on defense for any possible counterattacks. Let your jab lead in front of your combinations. A jab thrown in front of an opponent's face will block their vision briefly.

Always switch up the number of jabs thrown.

CHAPTER 17

COMBINATIONS

Combinations should be thrown with speed and power. Be creative and witty as combinations are made to trick the mathematician. Many counterpunchers will count the number of punches in your combinations. This will let them know when it's the right time to counterattack. Keep your combinations unpredictable.

When throwing combinations your punches get faster and more powerful from beginning to the end due to momentum. Build combination stamina by practicing combinations regularly, adding more punches, and slightly switching patterns as you go. Don't expect to land every punch. Some may get blocked. However, stick to your routine.

When executing combinations, always implement your motor functions. Stay on your toes and distribute your weight with each punch. Make sure you step with your jab and twist your torso and hips with your hooks and crosses. Keep your knees and hips slightly bent as you sit into your punches. Stand into your uppercuts.

Always keep your head moving. When throwing the left jab, as your torso twists to the right your head should slip to the right. When throwing the right cross, your torso should twist left as your head slips left.

"Let them feel your hands when you get a chance".

- Muhamin

CHAPTER 18

FIGHTING COMBINATIONS

Get creative and witty when creating combinations. Practice until it's second nature before you move on to the next combination. Combinations should be performed with speed and power. Constantly switch up your combinations to keep your opponent on edge.

These combinations are described in orthodox stance (left foot leading). If southpaw (right foot leading) switch left hand for right and right for left. Combinations should always be three strikes or more. The more the merrier.

Some combos to practice:

Double jab + Right hook body + Left hook head + Sidestep out.

Jab + Right cross body + Left hook body + Left uppercut head + Pivot step out.

Right cross head + Left hook head + Right hook body + Right hook head + Backstep with jab.

Right cross head + Jab + Right uppercut head + Left hook head + Pivot step out.

Double jab + Right cross head + Left hook body + Left hook head + Jab + Right cross + Pedal step out.

Triple jab + Right uppercut body + Right uppercut head + Left hook head + Right overhand head + Backstep with jab.

Jab body + Right cross body + Left uppercut head + Right hook head + Pivot step + Right hook body + Right hook head + Pedal step out.

Jab body + Double jab head + Right cross head + Pivot + Left uppercut + Right hook head + Double jab head + Sidestep out.

Right cross head + Left hook head + Right hook body + Left hook body + Left uppercut head + Right cross head + Backstep with jab.

Jab body + Double jab head + Right cross body + Double jab head + Right cross head + Jab + Right hook head + Left hook body + Left hook head + Right overhand head + Backstep out with jab.

CHAPTER 19

SHOULDER ROLL

The shoulder roll, like the uppercut, is a senior move or professional move in the sense that it must be perfected before use. Improper use of the shoulder roll can lead to you getting knocked out or ending up with a broken jaw.

The shoulder roll is simply using your leading shoulder to deflect the right or left cross. You can come back with a right or left cross of your own (a counterpunch).

Example:

Assuming the orthodox stance, your opponent shoots the left jab. You parry with the right hand. Then your opponent shoots the right cross. In your sideways pose, chin tucked, use your left shoulder to deflect your opponent's right cross by twisting to your body to the right side.

Shoulder rolls should be performed with your leading shoulder only. Roll to the right side, then shoot back a right cross, hook, or uppercut of your own.

CHAPTER 20

COUNTERPUNCH

A counterpuncher is the most feared boxer because you do not want to attack him. Every time you swing, he will make you pay. The only way to beat a counterpuncher is to also be a counterpuncher.

A counterpuncher has an exceptional defense, so much so that he will manipulate your offense. However, a counterpuncher can be predictable, in the sense that when you throw a punch, you know the open shot he's aiming for. An excellent counter puncher is a master at timing, so watch the shoulders.

The counter for a left jab can be a right-side step with a left hook, then slip right with a right-hand body blow or a slip with an uppercut. This is to be executed in one swift motion.

The counter for a right cross can be a left sidestep with a right hook, a slip left with a left-hand body blow, or once perfected, a shoulder roll with an added right cross.

The counter for a hook is a duck or a roll with a body blow, either a hook or jab.

CHAPTER 21
SHADOW BOXING

This is where you take everything that you have learned and put it all together. Use a mirror or record yourself to dot your i's and cross your t's. Head down, eyes up, chin tucked against your shoulder. Your body should follow your feet at a 45-degree angle. Slightly bend at the hips and knees, putting yourself in a slight sitting position. Stay up on the ball of your feet, keeping your heel raised.

Shadowboxing is an exercise and should be performed with the intensity of an actual fight. Practice makes permanent. Shadowboxing should be performed at full potential. Speed and power. This will build your endurance to fight stronger for longer.

Be sure to exercise head movement, footwork, and combinations.

CHAPTER 22

PAD WORK

"Boards don't hit back!"

-Bruce Lee

Pad work allows someone to train for offense and defensc in front of another person. Pad work is a step before sparring. It allows you to put your combinations together, and practice your slips, ducks, and rolls, all while exercising your footwork in front of a live human being.

Besides using the double-end bag, pad work is probably the best method to train hand-eye coordination in the boxing gym. Focus mitts usually come with a white circle, silver dollar size, in the center of the mitt.

Aim for the circle with your protruding knuckle.

CHAPTER 23

SPARRING

To spar is to fight for practice.

That being said, sparring is for learning only. Sparring is the last step before you actually compete. This is where you put everything that you have learned into action on another person.

Sparring should always be off-matched and monitored.

Example:

Amateur vs. professional. The pro will keep a level of professionalism in the ring while sharpening the amateur's craft. Sparring with an amateur will allow the pro to experiment with new theories and work on weaknesses.

Two amateurs cannot learn from each other, it's like the blind leading the blind. Two pros will just end up sizing each other up and fighting. Always mismatched for the best learning experience.

Sparring is the best preparation in training for a fight.

CHAPTER 24

REPETITION

"Practice makes permanent."

In his book, *Mastery*, Robert Greene says that 10,000 hours of practice is needed to reach a high level of skill in any craft. That's equivalent to seven to ten years of sustained solid practice. In boxing, 100 hours of training is needed for one minute of fighting.

For that reason, a fighter of any sport or art should know better than to play fight. 100 hours of training for an hour a day is equivalent to three months and ten days, just to fight for one minute. When play fighting, you're teaching yourself to not go hard and to not make full contact. You're actually deconditioning yourself.

Remember the five P's; Proper Preparation Prevents Poor Performance.

Make your technique second nature.

<h1 style="text-align:center">CHAPTER 25</h1>

STRATEGY

"If you fail to plan, then you must plan to fail."

With that being said, plan the fight in your head. This will give you the ability to be creative and visualize every aspect of your victory.

Visualize each step. Visualize your posture. Plan each combination and what's going to come next. Plan your defense. Be creative but realistic, and always be first.

If your opponent is much bigger than you are, visualize your victory by way of speed. If your opponent is much faster and smaller than you are, visualize the victory by way of strength and dominance. Seldom are fights evenly matched. In this case, plan the victory with craftiness.

Be skillfully tricky.

CHAPTER 26

FIGHTING STRATEGIES

Practice sparring one round of only defense. Another round of only jabs and footwork. A round of all combinations, and a round of only counterpunching.

Aim for the top of your opponent's biceps, just underneath the front shoulder muscle. When hit correctly, this will numb the arm and prevent your opponent from being able to lift his arm at you.

When striking the jawline, or sending a body blow to the rib cage, strike with your protruding knuckle, the back of your hand facing upward. Most people strike with their hand sideways, called a hammer fist. You will make contact with both the top and bottom jaw but never break anything. Position the backside of your hand facing upward, knuckles aligned with the single rib or the bottom jawline, and knock it off its hinges.

A shot to the bridge of the nose leaves two instant black eyes.

A twist of your fist when making contact with an eye will cut the eyelid.

If an opponent's hands are faster than yours, body blows can slow them down.

"Never duck the uppercut"

-   Tupac Shakur.

When fighting close contact on the inside, uppercuts to the body and head are most effective.

When parrying a punch, always go downward never upward.

When an opponent has his hands close to his face, pop a jab at his hand making him hit his own face. This will make him lower his hands.

Training with light hand weights, between one and three pounds, will make your hands faster, and light ankle weights will make your feet faster.

Forearm strengthening will make your fist tighter and harder and will strengthen your blocking.

Shoulder strengthening will make your punches stronger and give you knock-out power.

Strong calves will keep you on your toes throughout the fight.

Strong legs keep you from getting knocked down and helps you to sit on your punches.

A fake-out in front of a combination works like a charm.

Leading with a non-jab strike in the middle of a fight can confuse an opponent.

Set the tone. Pop first.

Never duck nor roll with your head down.
Shadowbox with the intensity of a brawl.

CHAPTER 27

MAKE THEM MISS BY CENTIMETERS

The science of boxing is to hit an opponent while making them miss. No one in their right mind likes to be hit. However, the answer is not to dodge the punch, but to simply evade it. Make an experienced fighter miss by a mile and they will surely switch the punch to something more effective. Make an opponent miss by centimeters and watch as they return with the same punch or combination. This will give you time to put together a counterpunch of your own.

CHAPTER 28

RECORD YOURSELF

We are our own worst critics. We often find flaws in ourselves that no one else sees. Use this as a method to fine-tune your craft. For years, fighters used mirrors to correct their mistakes, but we are now in the technological era. The ability to record lets you replay and document your mistakes. Learn from them!

Record training sessions, sparring sessions, and fights.

CHAPTER 29

PRACTICE IN THE SHADOWS

Train during off-peak gym hours as often as possible. This will provide more one-on-one time with your trainer, a less crowded environment, more free access to equipment, and fewer eyes on your technique. This will make your technique appear effortless and new because nobody was there to witness the long hours and preparation it took to perfect it.

Training in the shadows will also prevent other fighters from figuring out your style. Potential opponents may be watching.

CHAPTER 30

NEVER FIGHT A SPARRING PARTNER

Usually sparring partners train at the same gym. They might be friends or acquaintances. This creates a big brother/little brother effect. Trainers have different methods for choosing sparring partners for their fighters. Sparring partners are evenly matched to check one's capabilities. They may be outmatched to sharpen skills, or under-matched to practice theory. Your sparring partner will get familiar with all of your strengths and weaknesses. Challenging a sparring partner to a fight will be like staging an uneven match.

Example:

Roy Jones Jr. vs. Antonio Tarver.

Sparring is not a fight. It is a learning session. One that is meant for practice and gaining fighting experience.

CHAPTER 31
NEVER UNDERESTIMATE OPPONENTS

Ever heard the expression "Lucky Punch"? This is when the out-classed opponent lands a blow that ends the fight in his favor.

"Never judge a book by its cover."

What a person looks like has nothing to do with their skill set or knowledge.

Go into every fight with a strategy, and if by chance you should lose, let it be that you were outmatched, not that you underestimated your opponent.

Everyone is a potential threat!

CHAPTER 32

STAY CALM

The act of being anxious, angry, or excited, will leave you fatigued in a fight.

Stay calm! Think about what it is that you want to achieve and how you are going to go about it.

Stay calm! There is a much-needed conversation that should be going on silently in your head. A conversation where you are telling yourself that you got this. To stay relaxed. To pace yourself. A conversation where you inform yourself mentally, step by step of your strategy.

Remain Calm!

CHAPTER 33

STAY HUMBLE

Arrogance breeds humility! The time that one spends bragging and boasting, another person spends training. Being humble is an act of discipline and patience that will open far more opportunities than arrogance. Arrogance comes from a feeling of completion or a state of superiority. A true knuckle technician knows that there is always more to learn and areas that can use more development.

Never brag. Let your work speak for itself.

CHAPTER 34

BUILD YOUR OWN STYLE

Once you have mastered the fundamentals and learned which punches work well for you, you should then begin to put together a strategy of your own.

Study the great fighters and practice what it was that made them great. Adopt the style to your own and perfect it.

Example:

Muhammad Ali's footwork. Roy Jones Jr.'s defense. Mike Tyson's offense.

Perfect a style and own it.

CHAPTER 35

HEART

In the fight game, winners are usually the ones who want it the most. This is called heart. Refusal to fail. Refusal to quit. Always pushing yourself harder. As they say, "It's not the size of the dog in the fight, it's the size of the fight in the dog." Find something worth fighting for and use it as motivation to never give up.

CHAPTER 36

TACTIC'S OF A WINNER

One should learn how to defend himself before one learns how to attack someone.

My observation from watching fights is that the fighter who utilizes footwork usually wins.

It has been said that the one who does his road work will do what he wants in the fight, and the one who does not will do what he can.

Speed will give you the ability to whip an opponent, while strength will give you the ability to quickly end a fight.

When in a fight stay active. Go in cold. Leave out cold.

Keep your head moving.

Keep your hands up.

Stay on your toes.

Always show heart. Always have confidence.

CHAPTER 37

AUTHOR'S INSIGHT

Who's big enough to bring boxing back?

In the days of "Iron" Mike Tyson and Muhammad Ali, the streets were empty when they fought. Everyone was somewhere tuned in. Now it's all about mixed martial arts, but I'll say this:

Fight me like a man!

Growing up, when I fought my older sister, she would kick all sense out of me. Her kicks hurt and were effective. However, I was fighting a female. I'm also not interested in being mounted by a man the same way I make love to a female. So again, I say:

Fight me like a man!

My statement is this: Is there anyone brave enough to bring boxing back? Man to man. Hand to hand. Who will be the next great? The crime rate is rising due to gun violence. Where are all the knuckle technicians at? Don't get me wrong, I'm not against any art form as a means to a solution. But again, I say:

Fight me like a man!

CHAPTER 38

NUTRITION

Always consult a certified nutritional specialist first. Everyone's body is different, so what's good for me may not work for you. The following is basic information and nutrition that I use personally. I am not a certified nutrition specialist!

- A banana before and after each workout.

- Vitamin B for energy.

- Vitamin E for a healthy heart and cardiovascular system.

- A multivitamin for overall health.

- Protein powder for muscle health.

- Amino acid to break down your proteins.

- Plenty of water. Water distributes the nutrients throughout your body.

CHAPTER 39

BOXING WORKOUTS

Warm-up: Stretch all of your muscles for 10-15 minutes.

Jumping Jacks: 100 count.

Speed Bag: Three rounds for three minutes each round.

Heavy Bag: Six rounds for three minutes each round, or twice as many rounds intended to fight.

Row Rope: Three rounds for three minutes each round.

Focus Pads: Four rounds for three minutes each round.

Double-end bag: Four rounds for three minutes each round, or twice as many rounds intended to fight.

Sparring: Six rounds for three minutes each round, or twice as many rounds intended to fight. Use multiple partners.

Shadowboxing: Four rounds for three minutes each round. Alternate with the jump rope. Move around.

Jump Rope: Five rounds for three minutes each round. Alternate with shadowboxing. Move around.

CHAPTER 40
CALISTHENIC WORKOUT

Pull-ups: 10 sets of 10 reps

Bar Dips: 10 sets of 15 reps

Push-ups: 200 to 400 reps

Squats: 10 sets of 10 reps

Lunges: Four sets of 20 steps

Calf Raises: Four sets of 50 raises

Bunny Hops: Two sets of 30 hops

Duck Walks: Two sets of 30 steps

Leg Lifts: Four sets of 25 reps

Sit-ups: Four sets of 25 reps

Crunches: Two sets of 50 reps

Scissor Kicks: Two sets of 30 reps

Flutter Kicks: Two sets of 30 reps

Bicycles: Two sets of 40 reps

Sit-up Twists: Two sets of 20 reps

CHAPTER 41

CARDIO

Jogging: One hour or four miles at minimum.

Sprinting: 100-yard dashes. Work your way up to 10 sets.

Jumping Jacks: Two to three sets of 100.

Jump rope: 30 to 45 minutes.

Jogging in Place: Four sets for one minute each. Knees up high.

Pick a sport to participate in.

ABOUT THE AUTHOR

My name is Joseph Johnson, better known as Bruza. I was born on the 19th of May 1982. Fond of boxing since day one, I like to believe that boxing chose me. I grew up on movies like *One Armed Boxer*, the first five *Rocky* movies, and *Gladiator* with Cuba Gooding Jr.

I've been slap boxing and fist-fighting since elementary school. The middle child of four siblings, I often fought a lot at home, as well as in the streets.

The first boxing gyms I stepped into were Saint Mary's Recreation Center and Betances Recreation Center, located on 146th Street and Saint Ann's Avenue. I was in junior high school and moving from the South Bronx to the North East Bronx, so I could only attend these recreational centers on the weekends. That meant my training was limited and short-lived, and at that time I did not adapt to boxing fundamentals.

In 1997, I was enrolled in Samuel L. Gompers High School and attended the first half of the semester as a sophomore. That semester I got into an altercation, one which I couldn't avoid. This led to me being expelled due to the injuries of my opposition. I was arrested and banned from school grounds. This altercation is what got me the name Joe Bruiser.

My arresting officer didn't believe that I caused those injuries with my hand. He referred me to a boxing gym just off of Third Avenue on 150th Street called Jerome's Boxing Gym.

At that time, I was 15 years old, with no funds to pay for gym fees. The owner at that time knew my arresting officer, so he allowed me to sit in and watch. A few weeks later, my mother signed custody rights over to my aunt, and I was shipped off to live in Copiague, New York.

The third and final time I ran away from Long Island was when I was 17 years old. Only two weeks back in the Bronx and I already had a brush with the law on 86th Street in Manhattan. That landed me on juvenile probation and back into my mother's custody. I was mandated by the judge to attend my zone school for daily attendance, which was Evander Childs High School.

At Evander, I reunited with an old friend from Samuel L. Gompers. He told me about this boxing gym that was in the cut that no one knows about and suggested we go.

The gym was Morris Park Boxing Gym, and I believe that at the time the gym fees were $30 a month, and $20 a month for a trainer. My trainer's name was Tido. Back then I hated Tido. He made me train footwork for months. I wanted to hit the bag and spar. Today I wish Tido was in my corner.

My training at Morris Park only lasted for five months. I was expelled from Evander for fighting a security guard, and since I was living under my mother's roof, I was ordered to find a job.

From 2000 to 2006, I practiced wherever I could. I had the fundamentals down and all of my fighting experience came from the streets. Fighting in the streets kept me in bad situations. I was always going in and out of courtrooms.

A friend I knew from my neighborhood in the Edenwald Projects moved to the South Bronx near Prospect Avenue. He told me of a cheap gym near his house called Fort Apache Boxing Gym. I joined Fort Apache at the end of 2006 and was trained by the owner, Big George.

Big George instilled in me good technique. Punches in bunches. Hooks and uppercuts. Pivot and rolls. Big George told me that my money shots were going to be my left hook and right uppercut because he couldn't tell when they were coming out.

He made me practice combinations while rolling and pivoting under the straight rope. Minute drills for speed and the heavy bag for strength. Combinations and footwork on the heavy bag, and a lot of hooks and uppercuts to the bag on the wall. Big George only let me take advice and practice with the pros of the gym. Big ups to Sugar and his boy from Harlem.

At the end of 2007, everyone was talking about next year's Golden Gloves competition. Confident with my hand skills, I decided to sign up. I filled out and mailed in the application from *The Daily* newspaper. I was later called down to the Daily News Building on 34th Street where I took my physical, weighed in, and registered with the Boxing Association.

That night, I told everyone I knew that I was not only signed up but that I was coming home with my Golden Gloves. The Golden Gloves are a pendant one receives for winning the tournament.

About a week later, Big George announced that Fort Apache was being shut down. Fort Apache was an old gym that looked like an abandoned building. Chains to keep the doors close, the roof was missing pieces, there were cracks in the walls that led outside, and exposed pipes were everywhere.

A few fighters, along with myself, relocated to Jerome's Gym a block off of Third Ave. Big George was relocating there also. Jimmy, the owner of Jerome's Gym at the time, charged me the same price as Fort Apache, which was cheaper than his price.

Because of a conflict in schedule, I could no longer work with George. Big George worked in the mornings, and my job at the New York Sports Club led me to train in the afternoons and evenings. Jimmy decided to pick me up but refused to take me to the Golden Gloves tournament.

Jimmy's reasoning was that I've been working with Big George, and he did not want to disrespect and take credit for someone else's work, win or lose. Jimmy told me not to go to the Gloves that year because I would be going on my own, which is called going unattached. He said that unless I knocked everyone out, the judges would vote in favor of the gym. He told me to give him a year and he would guarantee me the gloves in 2009. But I made a promise to my peoples and decided to go anyway.

2008 rolled around, and I received a card in the mail welcoming me to the annual Golden Gloves tournament. I was to show up suited and ready to fight, at B.B. Kings on 42nd Street in Manhattan, a week from the date on the card.

Since the transfer to Jerome's Gym, Jimmy and I only trained defense. He told me, "Pride yourself on defense, all of the greats have amazing defense."

The week leading up to my first competitive fight I was introduced to a prison fighter/boxing coach named Yahya from the Albany Projects in Brooklyn. I was introduced to Yahya from a friend who was recently incarcerated with him.

It was the same friend from Gompers and Evander High School. At the meeting with Yahya, he informed me to stop jogging and to start sprinting and jumping rope for high impact. Yahya told me to shadowbox as if I were in a real fight. He taught me how to touch a man's soul. From that day on, I stopped punching and started stabbing my knuckles into my opponents. He also showed me how to cripple a man's offenses.

I wish I had more time to learn from Yahya, Insha'Allah, but we never met again.

Toward the middle of the week, I was at work sitting in my office when a co-worker brought me The Daily newspaper, showing me the Golden Gloves amateur welterweight contestants for the first bout of the year. I believe I was close to number eight. After seeing my name, Joseph Johnson, I was so excited that I screamed.

That afternoon my boy Muhamin called me for a sparring session, and I was going to accept all the help

I could get before I got in the ring. The training was intense. We were supposed to train for an hour and stayed for two or three hours.

The training started off with a workout. We then warmed up with shadowboxing and pad work, then finished with sparring. Before we knew it the gym had closed, and we were the last two left. That night we had made plans for Muhamin to be my cornerman.

The morning of the fight, I was sitting in my apartment stressed out. I needed black boxing shorts with no logo, a boxing cup, and boxing shoes. I begged but could not borrow the money to save my life.

Now I had my own boxing equipment, but it was not up to Golden Glove standards. Sports channels would be filming, so we couldn't advertise any logos. I think Everlast might have been acceptable. They wanted a professional-style boxing cup that covered your testicles, bladder, and kidneys. I believe the boxing shoes had to be a specific style also.

Don't quote me, but the fights may have started at 8 pm. Around 3 pm that afternoon, I got a call from my moms saying to come pick up the money for my equipment. I flew uptown, got the money, then flew to 28th Street in Manhattan to an Asian sporting goods store and purchased a cup, boxing shoes, and shorts. My items were over the amount of cash that I had. I explained my situation to the shop owner, and she let me have the items.

I jumped back on the train and reported straight to B.B. Kings on 42nd Street. I was one of the first fighters there. The place was empty. Slowly, guests and fighters poured in. All fighters were kept in the back, which looked like a basement.

I kept running to the bathroom to get a peek at the crowd as they were coming in. My boy Muhamin showed up, but when we walked to the back, we were told that he could not be my cornerman because I was listed as unattached and that one would be appointed to me. Muhamin returned to the guest area and I to the back.

I spoke to the other fighters, getting acquainted as we were being called one by one for the weigh-in. We sat in the back area waiting for what felt like hours waiting to be called. Everyone was talking about where they were from, what gym they trained at, and how long they've been training.

An announcement came over the speakers introducing the first two fighters. What were the chances? They not only called my name but the name of the fighter that I've been speaking to the entire time.

As we began to suit up, he was taken out because he didn't make weight. I was still called to the ring, and a new fighter by the name of Stouts was brought out to fight me. Walking from the backroom to the ring, my legs felt heavy, like bricks. At that moment, I had to pee and shit at the same time. My hand wraps felt too tight, and I wanted to back out.

We heard the screams from the crowd as they cheered us on. I walked up to the ring and ascended about four steps to the mat. As I stepped through the ropes and onto the mat, I kept telling myself, "Don't trip." The mat felt like stepping on a big sponge. I'm shown my corner as I wait for my opponent to step out.

Searching through the crowd with my eyes, I spot my family and friends. It looked like everybody came out. I was relieved, but still nervous because I never fought in front of so many people without getting in trouble for it.

My opponent stepped out; it was now my time. First fight of the year. First bout of the night. The crowd was screaming at us from all angles. Stout swung, sticking me on my headgear. At that moment all of my fears and worries went away.

Now we were fighting. As I look back, I displayed no skill in that fight. I only did what was natural to me at the time. However, I dropped Stouts in the 2nd and 3rd rounds and won by unanimous decision.

In its entirety, the outcome of the tournament was upsetting. Just as Jimmy stated, the decision was against me being unattached. I was voted against 2-1 in the semi-finals and lost. My opponent's coach and one of the female boxing officials came to me and told me that I really won the fight.

My opponent's coach told me that I need to get down with a gym, and that he would be willing to add me to his team. I declined. Angry and disappointed, I did not return to the gym that year. I began fighting in the streets and was shot that winter. Of all places to get hit, I got shot in my right arm.

It took a little over a year to heal an arm that doctors said would never work again. I suffered nerve damage, torn ligaments and tendons, and a fracture.

At the beginning of 2011, I returned to the gym. I found a spot called Main Street Boxing Gym in New Rochelle. This spot was nothing like the gyms I was used to. It was a flashier spot. However, we had plenty of sparring sessions. The owners took us to spar at Mount Vernon Boxing Gym, Kid Kelly's, and a few other places when we weren't sparring in-house.

I've been incarcerated serving an eight-year flat sentence since February 4, 2014. I get all my boxing done in the penile system. I even reunited with the fighter who didn't make his weight in my first fight.

My boxing techniques all come from trial and error through practice, experiment, and experience.

This book is not meant to turn you pro, but to teach you some of what I know.

THE END

We Help You Self-Publish Your Book
You're The Publisher and We're Your Legs!

Crystell Publications is not your publisher, but we will help you self-publish your own novel.

Ask About our Payment Plans

Crystal Perkins, MHR
Essence Magazine Bestseller
PO BOX 8044 / Edmond – OK 73083
www.crystellpublications.com
(405) 414-3991

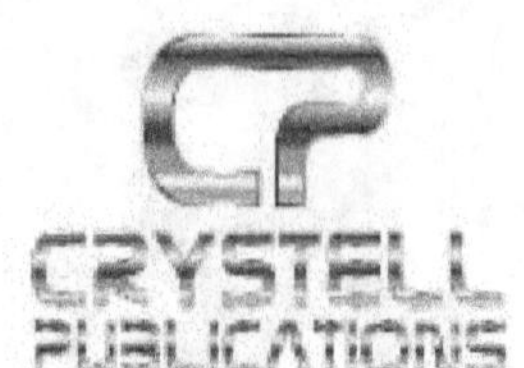

Plan 1-A 190 - 250 pgs. $699.00   **Plan 1-B 150 -180 pgs. $674.00**

Plan 1-C 70 - 145pgs $625.00

2 (Publisher/Printer) Proofs, Correspondence, 3 books, Manuscript Scan and Conversion, Typeset, Masters, Custom Cover, ISBN, Promo in Mink, 2 issues of Mink Magazine, Consultation, POD uploads. 1 Week of E-blast to a reading population of over 5000 readers, book clubs, and bookstores, The Authors Guide to Understanding The POD, and writing Tips, and a review snippet along with a professional query letter will be sent to our top 4 distributors in an attempt to have your book shelved in their bookstores or distributed to potential book vendors. After the query is sent, if interested, the distributors will contact you to discuss the shipment of your books and any fee

Plan 2-A 190 - 250 pgs. $645.00   **Plan 2-B 150 -180 pgs. $600.00**

Plan 2-C 70 - 145pgs $550.00

1 Printer Proof, Correspondence, 3 books, Manuscript Scan and Conversion, Typeset, Masters, Custom Cover, ISBN, Promo in Mink, 1 issue of Mink Magazine, Consultation, POD upload.

www.ingramcontent.com/pod-product-compliance
Lightning Source LLC
Chambersburg PA
CBHW050046260726
48658CB00005B/1809